Didja Know?

365

Surprising & Important

Health Facts

Bette Dowdell

DIDJA KNOW?
365 Surprising & Important Health Facts

published by
Confident Faith Institute LLC
PO Box 11744
Glendale AZ 85318

http://BetteDowdell.com

First Print Edition

ISBN#: 978-0-9889953-0-7

Bette Dowdell is not a medical professional of any sort; she is a patient who researched her way out of a very deep health ditch when professionals failed.

CONTENTS

http://BetteDowdell.com

INTRODUCTION

A month before my first birthday, a drunk driver smashed into my parents' car, I catapulted into the door face-first, and I lived with the consequences until I figured out how to fix the mess on my own. Doctors didn't seem to know how to help.

In my twenties, all signs indicated I would be checking out of this life shortly, but doctors still insisted I was fine, and I realized, as the saying goes, "If it is to be, it's up to me." And so my research—and my step-by-step journey to healing—began.

Years—and thousands of pages—later, searching for an elusive, missing piece of my puzzle, I was standing in line at the grocery store and saw a magazine cover screaming "Fix Your Adrenal Fatigue."

Well, I had whacked adrenal glands, not fatigued ones. But close enough. Any port in a storm—and other such sayings.

The article offered lots of information, most of which didn't fit. But one short sentence jumped out at me. I can't even remember what it said, just that it gave me a hook to help in my search.

Because of all it led me to, that one sentence made a huge difference in my health.

http://BetteDowdell.com

Some people call that sort of thing serendipity. Others call it dumb luck. I call it striking gold.

Didja Know: 365 Surprising and Important Health Facts has, as the title says, 365 health nuggets, one for each day of the year. While they won't all apply to everybody, many will. There's a good chance you, too, could strike gold.

You won't read these health facts in magazines. Or hear them in doctors' offices. And they sure aren't "conventional wisdom." They come from my years of research.

I found them, verified them and tried them. And now I offer them to you, hoping–and believing–they'll give your health the boost it needs.

A single sentence, of course, won't tell you everything you need to know. This book is about clues to help you on your way.

The first group of *Didja Knows* is about the endocrine system, a mystery to most people–a mystery we need to unravel. Why? The endocrine system controls our health, and believe you me, when the endocrine system ain't happy, ain't nothin' happy.

Then we stomp through Vitamins and Minerals, Herbs, Diet, Body Parts, Health Maladies, Drugs and Fluoride–with bits and pieces of things you should know.

Don't skip any *Didja Know*, even if you're absolutely convinced it has nothing to do with you. It could surprise you by being the clue you need.

It's like panning for gold; you can't predict where you'll find some nuggets.

The Resources chapter describes my other books and programs that give you detailed information about what's covered in this book.

If you want to read more of my story, you'll find it in the About Bette Dowdell chapter.

God is good,
Bette Dowdell
bette@BetteDowdell.com

("Bette" has two syllables. "Dowdell" rhymes with "cow bell.")

THE ENDOCRINE SYSTEM

Here we have the most complicated system known to mankind. Each part of the system has an appointed purpose, but they regularly get into each other's business—sometimes by design, other times because things get out of balance, and everybody on the team ends up bailing like crazy.

First, the parts of the system, with a word or so about their purpose:

Hypothalamus - Controls and coordinates the endocrine system and the nervous system

Pituitary - Controls the endocrine system, growth hormone, water balance, etc., etc., etc.

Thyroid - Energy and metabolism

Parathyroids - Keep calcium in balance

Adrenals - Energy and fight/flight

Pineal - Maintains our internal clock

Thymus - Immune system

Testes and *ovaries* - Estrogen, progesterone, testosterone

Pancreas - Blood sugar balance

http://BetteDowdell.com

Bones - Interacts with other endo glands, especially thyroid

Body fat - Creates hormones to control hunger

Now some endocrine *Didja Knows*.

1. Didja know the vastly misunderstood endocrine system controls our health?

2. Didja know if your thyroid's in trouble, the rest of your endocrine system going down?

3. Didja know when your endocrine system's in trouble, the rest of your health heads down a bad path? Where you end up is a "weakest link" thing.

4. Didja know thyroid tests are unreliable? The TSH test is the worst, but they're all a bad lot.

5. Didja know symptoms diagnose your thyroid status, not tests? And who knows your symptoms best?

6. Didja know docs rely only on tests to see what's up with the thyroid, so we're on our own?

7. Didja know no endocrine gland thrives or suffers alone? If one goes, the others follow.

8. Didja know if your thyroid takes down your pineal gland, sleep becomes a problem?

http://BetteDowdell.com

9.   Didja know if your thyroid takes down your thymus, there goes your immune system?

10.   Didja know your thyroid can take down your adrenals, a health disaster?

11.   Didja know if your thyroid interrupts your pancreas, your blood sugar goes whacky?

12.   Didja know low thyroid causes osteoporosis?

13.   Didja know low thyroid causes low stomach acid—and there goes the digestive system?

14.   Didja know a whacked endocrine system leads to turkey-trot digestion problems?

15.   Didja know a whacked endocrine system can lead to interstitial cystitis?

16.   Didja know an underactive thyroid doubles your chance of heart trouble?

17.   Didja know low thyroid causes low iron—and taking iron is the wrong answer?

18.   Didja know bromine, as in bread, etc., causes an underactive thyroid?

19.   Didja know fluoride murders the thyroid—along with other body parts?

http://BetteDowdell.com

20.   Didja know soy kills the endocrine system?

21.   Didja know mineral deficiencies whack the endocrine system big time?

22.   Didja know the endocrine system is a nutrition hog? Needs it. Demands it. Goes down without it.

23.   Didja know a low-fat diet drags the endocrine system into a dark pit?

24.   Didja know prostate cancer comes from too much estrogen?

25.   Didja know low thyroid and high cholesterol go together?

26.   Didja know progesterone is the Miss Congeniality of hormones?

27.   Didja know estrogen can be a witch on wheels and cause chaos throughout the body?

28.   Didja know testosterone is too much of a gentleman?

29.   Didja know nighttime use of CFL bulbs messes with the pineal gland?

30.   Didja know too much calcium can take out the parathyroid glands?

http://BetteDowdell.com

31.   Didja know an underactive thyroid makes it hard for your body to make new bone cells?

32.   Didja know endocrine function depends on good liver health?

33.   Didja know low thyroid causes sleep apnea?

34.   Didja know estrogen dominance, when estrogen runs wild, leads to breast cancer?

35.   Didja know mercury can cause thyroid problems?

36.   Didja know dental sealants usually contain endocrine-disrupting BPA? BPA is a form of estrogen.

37.   Didja know low testosterone can cause angina pain?

38.   Didja know diabetics have low thyroid function?

39.   Didja know frequent sighing is a sign of adrenal problems?

VITAMINS AND MINERALS

40.   Didja know people may be hungry all the time because of a magnesium deficiency?

41.   Didja know a vitamin B9 deficiency causes damage similar to radiation?

42.   Didja know a magnesium deficiency accelerates aging? .

43.   Didja know vitamin/mineral deficiencies cause sleep problems?

44.   Didja know Advil "works" by sucking up your copper?

45.   Didja know a solid vitamin/mineral program prevents/reverses an enlarged prostate?

46.   Didja know vitamin C reduces the risk of vaccine side-effects?

47.   Didja know calcium stiffens blood vessels, raising blood pressure?

48.   Didja know magnesium relaxes blood vessels and lowers blood pressure?

49.   Didja know the mineral boron increases alertness?

50.   Didja know a biotin deficiency can make you itchy?

51.   Didja know a thiamine deficiency can look like senility?

52.   Didja know chlorine destroys our thiamine (B1)?

53.   Didja know a riboflavin deficiency makes you light sensitive?

54.   Didja know a lack of riboflavin (B2) can lead to cancer?

55.   Didja know birth control pills shut out riboflavin (B2)?

56.   Didja know you need riboflavin (B2) to create healthy red blood cells?

57.   Didja know thyroid problems require extra riboflavin (B2)?

58.   Didja know a lack of niacinamide (one form of B3) makes you a lame brain?

59.   Didja know niacin (another form of B3) lowers blood fat levels?

60.   Didja know vitamin B6 prevents oxalate kidney stones?

61.   Didja know a high-carb diet destroys our chromium?

62.   Didja know good chromium levels improve the symptoms of diabetes?

http://BetteDowdell.com

63.   Didja know our bodies can't really absorb the
        carbonate form of calcium?

64.   Didja know magnesium oxide doesn't absorb as well
        as other forms of magnesium?

65.   Didja know a B12 deficiency can get misdiagnosed as
        Alzheimer's?

HERBS

66. Didja know the herb hawthorn heals damaged hearts?

67. Didja know 1/3 of us can't tolerate the widely touted herb, chlorella?

68. Didja know DHEA you take doesn't work like the DHEA our bodies make?

69. Didja know the herb boswellia helps with arthritic pain?

70. Didja know the herb hawthorn can ease anxiety?

71. Didja know the herb milk thistle protects your liver?

72. Didja know the noxious weed stinging nettle has seeds that help failing adrenals?

73. Didja know the herb boswellia can lower blood pressure?

74. Didja know the herb burdock can boost metabolism?

75. Didja know the herb milk thistle can shrink fibroids?

76. Didja know the herb garlic boosts the immune system's killer cells?

77.   Didja know steroid meds stomp all over testosterone?

78.   Didja know the horse chestnut herb fights varicose veins?

79.   Didja know the herb boswellia used to be known as frankincense? Been around a while.

80.   Didja know the great tasting herb anise helps breathing?

81.   Didja know the ancient herb ashwagandha can increase physical endurance?

82.   Didja know the herb astragalus boosts healing?

83.   Didja know the herb bilberry can correct night blindness?

84.   Didja know the herb borage helps endocrine balance?

85.   Didja know the herb cat's claw can help intestinal problems?

86.   Didja know the herb clove helps fight parasites?

87.   Didja know the herb feverfew combats muscle spasms?

88.   Didja know the herb ginger helps fight morning sickness?

89.   Didja know the herb yarrow helps heal mucous
        membranes?

90.   Didja know the herb parsley helps thyroid function?

91.   Didja know evening primrose oil heals dry eye?

92.   Didja know the herb turmeric protects the liver?

93.   Didja know the herb witch hazel works as a facial
        toner?

94.   Didja know the herb slippery elm helps Crohn's, etc?

95.   Didja know the herb suma boosts the immune
        system?

DIET

96.   Didja know good saturated fat is your friend? Notice the word "good."

97.   Didja know parsley has three times the vitamin C of an orange?

98.   Didja know coconut oil helps prevent heart disease?

99.   Didja know low-fat milk causes skin problems?

100.   Didja know low-fat milk interferes with ovary function?

101.   Didja know factory-farm milk includes pus? Yum! There's even a government allowance for it.

102.   Didja know low-fat milk is a disaster for your hormones?

103.   Didja know polyunsaturated fats cause dry eye?

104.   Didja know a low-carb diet improves acne?

105.   Didja know a low-fat diet ages the skin?

106.   Didja know a low-carb diet lessens MS symptoms?

107.   Didja know a low-salt diet leads to heart fatalities?

108.   Didja know a low-carb diet helps the liver?

109.   Didja know a low-fat diet leads to insulin resistance?

110.   Didja know a low-carb diet boosts insulin sensitivity?

111.   Didja know a low-carb diet burns calories more efficiently?

112.   Didja know not all calories are equal? We can count 'em up, but the total doesn't mean squat.

113.   Didja know a USDA food pyramid diet is hard on your health?

114.   Didja know a high-carb diet makes gout worse?

115.   Didja know a high-sat-fat/low-carb diet improves epilepsy symptoms?

116.   Didja know a good diet can prevent hearing loss?

117.   Didja know polyunsaturated fats in the diet cause cataracts?

118.   Didja know a high-sat-fat/low-carb diet reduces ocular pressure?

119.   Didja know moisturizers with glycerin dry the skin?

120.   Didja know toothpaste with glycerin encourages plaque?

http://BetteDowdell.com

121. Didja know aspartame is addictive?

122. Didja know aspartame really whacks people with multiple sclerosis? Well, everybody, but especially those with MS.

123. Didja know Resveratrol's made from moldy grape skins?

124. Didja know strawberries can prevent esophageal cancer? Vitamins and minerals do a better job, of course, but whatever floats your boat.

125. Didja know MSG can destroy our nerves' protective coating? .

126. Didja know HFCS during pregnancy can damage a girl baby's endocrine function?

127. Didja know high fructose corn syrup is murder on your liver?

128. Didja know today's fruits and veggies have little nutrition?

129. Didja know a low-fat diet leads to gall bladder problems?

130. Didja know a low-fat diet tells your body to store fat?

131. Didja know coconut oil fights MRSA?

132.   Didja know a low-fat diet increases your risk of cancer?

133.   Didja know a low-fat diet speeds up aging?

134.   Didja know a low-fat diet loses muscle, not fat?

135.   Didja know a low-fat diet means you can't absorb nutrition?

136.   Didja know a low-fat diet leads to depression? And makes depression worse?

137.   Didja know a low-fat diet damages your metabolism? It's fixable, but not without effort.

138.   Didja know a low-fat diet throws the endocrine system into an unbalanced tizzy?

139.   Didja know a low-fat diet can cause hyperthyroidism? Hypothyroidism, too. Either way, you lose.

140.   Didja know a low-fat diet, such as that promoted by the American Diabetic Association, increases insulin resistance?

141.   Didja know a low-fat diet can cause infertility?

142.   Didja know your body makes your hormones from the saturated fat you eat? Low fat means low hormones.

143.   Didja know a low-fat diet leads to gallstones? .

http://BetteDowdell.com

144.   Didja know a low-fat diet worsens Crohn's Disease?

145.   Didja know a low-fat diet raises cholesterol levels?

146.   Didja know a low-fat diet starves your brain?

147.   Didja know a low-fat diet leads to chronic disease?

148.   Didja know a low-fat diet can explain acne?

149.   Didja know a low-fat diet causes cravings?

150.   Didja know a wrong-fat diet (vegetable oils) is at least as bad as a low-fat diet?

151.   Didja know athletes die younger than couch potatoes?

152.   Didja know sugar beets are genetically modified and beat up on your DNA?

153.   Didja know feeding grain to cows makes their meat unhealthy?

154.   Didja know grocery store milk includes insulin-like growth factor, leading to cancers?

155.   Didja know apples get drowned in pesticides, which makes them unhealthy?

156.   Didja know grocery store potatoes won't sprout eyes? Too many chemicals.

157.   Didja know farmed fish has little nutritional value?
        Including farmed salmon.

158.   Didja know most food cans are lined with synthetic
        estrogen? Look for glass containers.

159.   Didja know grass-fed beef has more Omega 3 fat than
        wild-caught salmon?

160.   Didja know your brain is mostly saturated fat? No fat
        means no brain.

161.   Didja know the endocrine system makes all its
        hormones from saturated fat?

162.   Didja know a low-fat diet leads to dread diseases?

163.   Didja know we can't absorb nutrition from any meal
        that doesn't include fat?

164.   Didja know microwaved popcorn leads to pancreatic,
        testicular and liver cancer?

165.   Didja know caffeinated coffee is a top-notch
        antioxidant?

166.   Didja know caffeinated coffee contains dietary fiber?

167.   Didja know stevia is chock-a-block full of good
        nutrition?

168.   Didja know drinking water raises your blood pressure? Even more than coffee. Who knew?

169.   Didja know our bodies don't need carbs? Fat and protein, yes. Carbs, no.

170.   Didja know a loss of libido can be nature's way of suggesting you need better nutrition?

171.   Didja know low calorie diets get rid of muscle, not fat?

172.   Didja know MSG and soy feed cancer? Why would you want to do that?

173.   Didja know a vegan diet makes you toot?

174.   Didja know vegetable oils lead to all sorts of diseases?

175.   Didja know a good vitamin/mineral program can prevent cancer?

176.   Didja know vegetable oils skyrocket your heart attack risk?

177.   Didja know grapes are inherently moldy? Wine, too.

178.   Didja know wheat was genetically modified about 50 years ago?

179.   Didja know drinking grocery store milk leads to estrogen dominance?

180.   Didja know "all natural" means anything anybody
        wants it to mean?

181.   Didja know the "USDA Organic" label has big-time
        exceptions?

182.   Didja know fast food wrappers contain chemicals
        leading to cancer? If the food doesn't get you, the
        wrapper will.

183.   Didja hear the USDA is promoting MSG for weight
        loss? The possibility of an autoimmune disease isn't
        mentioned.

184.   Didja know you can't detox mercury well without
        adequate protein?

185.   Didja know a lack of protein causes anemia?

186.   Didja know eating microwaved food depletes
        hemoglobin levels?

187.   Didja know grocery-store milk is more tainted than
        tap water? Yum!

188.   Didja know pasteurization doesn't kill all the bad
        guys? Including viruses? Kills nutrition, though.

189.   Didja know a WW2 shortage of bread in Holland
        reduced childhood mortality to almost nothing?

190. Didja know gluten really whacks people with fibromyalgia?

191. Didja know artificial sweeteners bulk up belly fat?

192. Didja know aspartame encourages the onset of Type 2 diabetes?

193. Didja know microwaving olive oil ruins its nutritional value?

194. Didja know chewing on gum releases insulin?

195. Didja know much of Europe bans U.S. beef as unsafe?

196. Didja know diet builds muscle while exercise tones it?

197. Didja know cholesterol doesn't cause heart attacks, but statin drugs do?

198. Did know a low protein diet causes cellulite?

199. Didja know a low protein diet speeds up aging? Muscles wasting and sagging. Skin pruning up. Energy leaving town. How can this be called good?

http://BetteDowdell.com

BODY PARTS

200.   Didja know if your liver doesn't work well, neither does anything else?

201.   Didja know donating your left kidney leads to trouble. Right seems to be okay.

202.   Didja know Tylenol is a major cause of liver damage?

203.   Didja know vitamin deficiencies can cause congestive heart failure?

204.   Didja know high fructose corn syrup raises uric acid levels? Can you say gout?

205.   Didja know low stomach acid can cause rosaceae?

206.   Didja know low stomach acid is common, while high stomach acid is rare? It's the fact they have the same symptoms that's confusing.

207.   Didja know a hard, poochy belly often means your liver's in trouble?

208.   Didja know today's typical diet causes liver cirrhosis?

209.   Didja know low stomach acid means you can't digest protein? Which is a catastrophe.

210.   Didja know your spleen is part of your immune
        system?

211.   Didja know your appendix is also part of your immune
        system?

HEALTH MALADIES

212. Didja know candida is a fungus that causes major health problems?

213. Didja know the typical diet feeds candida?

214. Didja know candida causes celiac disease?

215. Didja know candida whacks thyroid function?

216. Didja know the right nutritional supplements can tame candida?

217. Didja know candida makes autism worse?

218. Didja know candida creates thyroid antibodies?

219. Didja know candida causes inflammation, which causes disease?

220. Didja know candida runs wild when sugar or, especially, high fructose corn syrup show up?

221. Didja know men who get PSA tests die at the same rate as men who don't?

222. Didja know brain plaques are more a symptom of Alzheimer's than a cause?

223.   Didja know coconut oil lessens Alzheimer symptoms significantly?

224.   Didja know sulfur helps detox mercury?

225.   Didja know cigarette smoke contains the heavy metal cadmium?

226.   Didja know candida and gluten intolerance go together?

227.   Didja know food sensitivities and interstitial cystitis go together? Not cause-and-effect, but co-conspirators.

228.   Didja know interstitial cystitis gets diagnosed as a urinary tract infection, but that's not the name of the game—or the treatment.

229.   Didja know chlorine sets your arteries up for plaque?

230.   Didja know vaccine guidelines put 5000mcg of aluminum in your baby by 18 months?

231.   Didja know fluoride plays a big role in a variety of cancers?

232.   Didja know doctors are now the third leading cause of death in the U.S.?

233.   Didja know an Italian court agreed the MMR vaccine causes autism? Other courts are starting to join in.

234.   Didja know prescription acid blockers mess with your brain?

235.   Didja know lowering stomach acid can lead to deadly diarrhea?

236.   Didja know American Society for Nutrition shills for Big Pharma? And you were wondering why our diets are a mess?

237.   Didja know cystic fibrosis patients need heavy-duty nutrition?

238.   Didja know vaccines include the active ingredient glutamate, which is toxic to the brain?

239.   Didja know vaccines include aluminum to "get the attention" of your immune system?

240.   Aluminum, of course, is a heavy metal we don't want in our bodies–no way, no how.

241.   Didja know over-the-counter antacids contain aluminum?

242.   Didja know there's no science behind vaccines, and you need to really jigger the research to "prove" they work.

243.   Didja know five annual flu shots, starting at age 55, doubles your risk of dementia?

http://BetteDowdell.com

244. Didja know antiseptic mouth wash can raise your blood pressure?

245. Didja know fluorescent light bulbs raise blood sugar levels?

246. Didja know a low salt diet raises your risk of heart disease? Death, too.

247. Didja know lyme disease can get misdiagnosed as multiple sclerosis?

248. Didja know compact fluorescent light bulbs cause fatigue?

249. Didja know hormone-disrupting phthalates are used in breast implants?

250. Didja know WebMD.com speaks for Big Pharma? It's about money, honey.

251. Didja know you can't sue vaccine manufacturers, no matter what damage they cause, because the government gives them a free pass.

252. Didja know women with high cholesterol live longer, healthier lives?

253. Didja know osteoporosis drugs weaken bones? They look thick, but snap like twigs.

254.   Didja know cholesterol doesn't cause heart
        problems? Inflammation does.

255.   A healthy cholesterol level is between 200 and 300.
        Yeah, I know that's not what the doc told you, but it's
        true.

256.   Didja know caramel coloring begets inflammation–the
        start of all disease?

257.   Didja know caramel coloring leads to insulin
        resistance–and Type 2 diabetes?

258.   Didja know aspartame can cause the same symptoms
        as multiple sclerosis. Usually reversible–once you
        ditch the aspartame.

http://BetteDowdell.com

DRUGS

259.   Didja know Coumadin can cause osteoporosis and/or heart disease?

260.   Didja know a side effect of statin drugs is irritability?

261.   Didja know cholesterol-lowering drugs can cause heart disease?

262.   Didja know the recommended diabetes diet makes things worse? Wrong diet.

263.   Didja know diabetes drugs can cause heart attacks?

264.   Didja know diet is more effective in healing diabetes than prescription drugs?

265.   Didja know fluoride-based antibiotics such as Cipro can cause tendon damage?

266.   Didja know antidepressants increase breast cancer risk?

267.   Didja know antibiotics raise your risk of death? Hard on the immune system, don't you know.

268.   Didja know bariatric surgery guarantees significant vitamin/mineral deficiencies?

269.   Didja know antibiotics increase breast cancer risk?

270. Didja know antidepressants don't fix anything; vitamins and minerals do. In spades.

271. Didja know statin drugs cause diabetes?

272. Didja know statin drugs lead to congestive heart failure?

273. Didja know statin drugs damage your liver?

274. Didja know CoQ10 (ubiquinol) helps protect your liver from statins?

275. Didja know statin drugs increase your risk of Parkinson's Disease?

276. Didja know hormone replacement treatment (HRT) shrinks the brain?

277. Didja know aspirin increases your risk of "wet" macular degeneration?

278. Didja know nonsteroidal anti-inflammatories (NSAID) increase your risk of internal bleeding?

279. Didja know T4 meds, such as Synthroid, don't actually treat hypothyroidism? Make the tests look good, though.

FLUORIDE

280. Didja know fluoride is murder on the endocrine system?

281. Didja know fluoride beats up your digestive system?

282. Didja know fluoride eats collagen, inviting wrinkles galore? Yikes!

283. Didja know fluoride causes tendon damage? A known side-effect of newer antibiotics.

284. Didja know fluoride sucks all the moisture from your skin?

285. Didja know fluoride is hard on the liver? Really, really hard.

286. Didja know fluoride causes inflammation, which then causes disease.

287. Didja know fluoride weakens teeth?

288. Didja know nearly half the kids in the U.S. have mottled teeth from fluoride?

289. Didja know fluoride lowers kids' IQs? Doesn't do anything good for adult brains, either.

290. Didja know fluoride drains your emotions so you don't care?

291.   Didja know fluoride eats your bones? Yeah, I know
        that's not what you read.

292.   Didja know fluoride worsens the symptoms of
        autism?

293.   Didja know fluoride increases your chances of a heart
        attack?

294.   Didja know fluoride causes autoimmune diseases?

295.   Didja know fluoride causes hypothyroid symptoms by
        the carload?

296.   Didja know fluoride drains your energy?

297.   Didja know fluoride causes learning problems?

298.   Didja know fluoride makes your body temperature
        fluctuate?

299.   Didja know fluoride causes diabetes?

300.   Didja know fluoride causes gum disease?

301.   Didja know fluoride causes joint pain?

302.   Didja know fluoride causes heart palpitations?

303.   Didja know fluoride causes depression?

304.   Didja know fluoride causes chest pains?

305.   Didja know fluoride causes dizziness?

306.   Didja know fluoride causes sleep problems?

307.   Didja know fluoride causes shortness of breath?

308.   Didja know fluoride causes restlessness?

309.   Didja know fluoride causes thirst?

310.   Didja know fluoride causes tinnitus?

311.   Didja know fluoride messes with your eyesight?

312.   Didja know fluoride whacks the body's 24-hour clock?

313.   Didja know fluoride increases light sensitivity?

314.   Didja know fluoride causes nausea?

315.   Didja know fluoride leads to strokes?

316.   Didja know fluoride flushes out magnesium—which we need for more than 300 internal functions?

317.   Didja know fluoride lowers yet-to-be-born kids' IQs during pregnancy if Mom drinks or bathes in it?

318.   Didja know fluoride weakens teeth?

319.   Didja know fluoride weakens tendons and makes them easier to tear?

320.   Didja know fluoride causes hypothyroidism?

321.   Didja know fluoride plays a role in chronic fatigue syndrome?

322.   Didja know negative research results on fluoride get censored—with your tax dollars?

323.   Didja know every single claim of fluoride's benefits is bogus?

324.   Didja know fluoride ages your skin big time?

325.   Didja know fluoride makes you susceptible to hip fracture?

326.   Didja know dentists in fluoridated areas earn more money than those working in non-fluoridated areas?

327.   Didja know fluoride causes stiff joints?

328.   Didja know fluoride contributes to COPD?

329.   Didja know fluoride blocks vitamin B3, needed for our energy cycle?

330.   Didja know fluoride plays a big role in bone cancer?

331.   Didja know fluoride plays a big role in liver cancer?

332.   Didja know chronic fluoride poisoning causes fibromyalgia?

333.   Didja know areas with fluoridated water have the
       highest rate of obesity?

334.   Didja know many meds contain a extra potent form
       of fluoride?

335.   Didja know fluoride is as toxic as arsenic?

336.   Didja know fluoride creates nutritional deficiencies?

337.   Didja know fluoride creates tons of free radicals to
       rust out your body parts?

338.   Didja know a magnesium deficiency makes you more
       susceptible to fluoride?

339.   Didja know Harvard researchers classify fluoride with
       mercury?

340.   Didja know fluoride crosses the placenta and attacks
       the baby?

341.   Didja know long-term effects of fluoride have never
       been studied?

342.   Didja know fluoride poisoning can get diagnosed as
       Alzheimer's?

343.   Didja know your tax dollars pay for the fluoride that
       destroys your health?

344.   Didja know fluoride trashes your immune system?

http://BetteDowdell.com

345.   Didja know fluoride increases your risk of diabetes?

346.   Didja know fluoride causes interstitial cystitis?

347.   Didja know Nestle's bottled water is fluoridated?

348.   Didja know fluoride causes cancer? Breast, prostate, whatever.

349.   Didja know the fluoride they put in our water is industrial waste?

350.   Didja know fluoride causes crowded teeth?

351.   Didja know fluoride causes bone cancer?

352.   Didja know fluoride causes bladder cancer?

353.   Didja know fluoride turns normal cells into cancer cells?

354.   Didja know fluoride increases your need for sleep?

355.   Didja know fluoride causes early menopause?

356.   Didja know fluoride causes early puberty?

357.   Didja know fluoride causes diarrhea?

358.   Didja know fluoride deactivates your thyroid, but tests can't tell?

359. Didja know the fluoride they add to our water is industrial waste?

360. Didja know fluoride feeds candida?

361. Didja know fluoride thins your hair? Who thinks that's a good idea?

362. Didja know fluoride's hard on fingernails? Weak, ridged and short.

363. Didja know fluoride depletes your body's health-producing glutathione?

364. Didja know fluoride is hard on ADHD?

365. Didja know Coca Cola contains fluoride?

RESOURCES

Too Pooped to Participate is a free, weekly e-newsletter containing health information you probably won't hear about anyplace else.

http://TooPoopedToParticipate.com

Your Key to Good Health: The Amazing Endocrine System lists the parts of the endocrine system, describes what each does and how to tell if they're not doing it all that well. It's available from Amazon either for the Kindle or as a paperback book.

http://budurl.com/EndoSystem

Understanding Blood Tests is a downloadable e-book that describes eight common blood tests and explains the results. Everybody needs four of the tests, while the other four are more situational.

http://UnderstandBloodTests.com

Moving to Health is a 52-week program that explains how your body works, what makes it not work and what to do about it. Everything connects to everything in our bodies, so that's an important part of what's covered. And, of course, what our symptoms are telling us. We need to become our own health advocates, and *Moving To Health* leads the way.

http://MovingToHealth.com

BetteDowdell.com is the place to go for links to everything I do.

http://BetteDowdell.com

ABOUT BETTE DOWDELL

A month before my first birthday, while driving down the highway to Grandpa and Grandma's house for Christmas, a drunk driver smashed into my parents' car.

In those days before seat belts were mandated, our little car had none.

My mother smashed through the windshield, then bounced back, her face hitting the dashboard—where she left her perfect teeth embedded. She suffered a traumatic brain injury, from which she never fully recovered—although doctors proclaimed her to be as fit as a fiddle.

My father hit the steering wheel with his ribs and the dashboard with his knees. While he couldn't walk for a while, he recovered.

Fortunately, my brothers (7 and 5 years old) and sister (not quite 3) were protected because they were playing on the floor in the back seat—which my father had suggested just moments before, to limit their energetic activities a bit.

I torpedoed, face first, from my mother's lap into the car door. The impact tore all the skin from my forehead, and I suffered a concussion.

Doctors didn't know (many still don't) that most concussions damage the pituitary gland, which controls the endocrine system, which, in turn, controls all of health. (Another thing doctors don't seem to know.)

According to the docs, I was fine—within minutes after the crash, in fact.

But my mother realized something was wrong.

And so started my doctor visits, each of which ended with the verdict I was fine, followed by a little sermonette for my mother about not making a mountain out of a mole hill, as the saying goes.

But God bless my mother. She kept trying. (Note to doctors: Believe the mother.)

We moved a lot, so a new town meant new doctors, and maybe one of them would help. But, no.

Meanwhile, as the "She's fine" chorus continued, my health slipped away. By my early twenties, I was in very deep trouble.

For one thing, my brain became undependable. While teaching computer programming at IBM, I would suddenly, mid-sentence, forget why I was in the room. Given the army of people staring at me as I stood in front of the room alone, I was obviously teaching, but what?

I couldn't hold on to a thought. Speaking became a chore because I couldn't come up with the words I needed. Most of my hair fell out, and what was left changed color. I couldn't stay awake. I answered the phone in my sleep and never knew it.

My blood pressure was 70/40. My blood sugar was 46. My body temperature was 95–on a good day. My pulse was in the fifties. I had Raynaud's Syndrome. And on, and on and on.

Doctors still said I was fine. One doctor suggested my problem was I wanted to get married. Another suggested my difficulties came from emotional problems he was sure all preacher's kids suffered. (I was too brain-dead to ask what problem all doctors' kids suffered.)

Finally, at long last, I found a doctor who took me seriously. One who had enough clout to do the right thing, whether or not it was the accepted answer. And internationally recognized for his diagnostic skills. WooHoo!

After several long office visits and more tests than I knew there were tests, he told me I had panhypopituitarism, which meant every part of my endocrine system was in a world of hurt. He started treatment, and life began picking up–when we moved across the country.

I ended up with "You're fine!" doctors again, and I realized it was up to me. Okay, I can do this–especially with a diagnosis to guide my search.

But I couldn't do it quickly. It's hard to find information that contradicts what medicine wants you to know. The research may be fabulous, but if the conclusion offends the poobahs, under the carpet it goes.

It took me more than thirty years to put the pieces together. I'm still digging around in the research, especially since the internet is setting free some solid research that's been buried for fifty or more years.

I learned:
- How the endocrine actually works, what makes it not work and what makes it work better.

- Our bodies falter without good nutrition—which turns out to be different from what we're told is good nutrition. So I studied a lot about nutrition—and found it improved my health even more than medicines.

- We're surrounded by enemies—toxins in the air and water, toxic artificial ingredients in our food, genetically-modified foods that do enormous harm to our DNA, and more. So I studied a lot about toxins. We can't get rid of all toxins, but we can lighten the load, which gives good nutrition the help it needs to win the battle.

So that's the stuff I write about.

Along with a 500-pound gorilla nobody talks about: Getting diagnosed. Diagnosing health problems is a lost art.

http://BetteDowdell.com

Nowadays, doctors are required to diagnose via simple blood tests—many of which are unreliable. Maybe even most.

The doctor who diagnosed my pituitary problem used tests—some simple, some very advanced—not to diagnose, but to support his analysis of my symptoms. That doesn't happen any more. I couldn't get diagnosed nowadays.

But without a diagnosis, how can we know what to do?

It's about symptoms—as it always has been.

Symptoms tell the story of your health. They are your body's way of telling you what's going on. And who knows your symptoms better than you? So I point out what symptoms mean what.

By putting together my information about symptoms, nutrition, toxins, etc., you can figure out where you are—and what you can do to move to a better place.

That's how I got out of the ditch. And you don't have to trudge through thirty years of research to follow along. Good, eh?

Our bodies do amazing things when we give them the help they need.

http://BetteDowdell.com

INDEX

www.ingramcontent.com/pod-product-compliance
Lightning Source LLC
Chambersburg PA
CBHW060644280326
41933CB00012B/2149